CW00469483

VEGAN & GLUTEN-FREE
COOKBOOK
OF
AMERICAN
FAVOURITES

AMERICAN COOKING WITHOUT COMPROMISE

Annette Heringmann

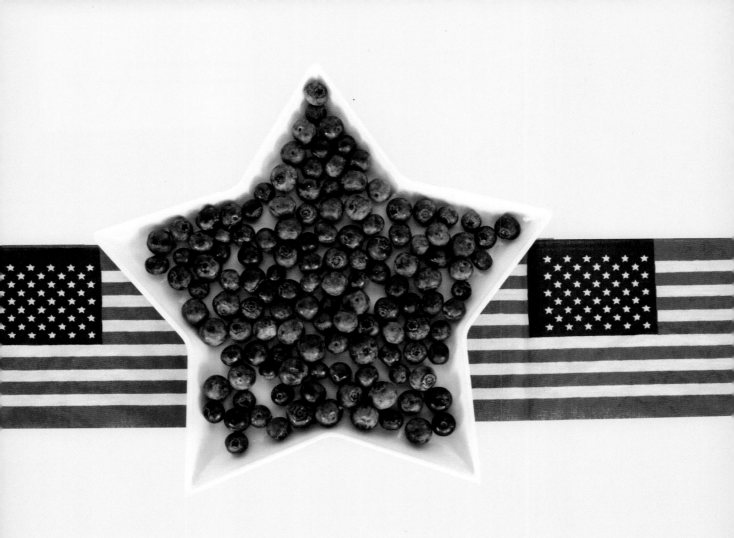

COPYRIGHT © 2020 ANNETTE HERINGMANN

ALL RIGHTS RESERVED.

ISBN: 978-1-7770099-5-3

TABLE OF CONTENTS

TABLE OF CONTENTS

FOREWORD

When it comes to eating "American style", the thought of fast food or microwave dishes may come to mind. Such a simplistic view ignores the rich history of American cooking. A history that includes the colonial era followed by waves of immigration from the four corners of the world. When the British, Dutch, and French arrived in the New World, they brought with them their dishes, ingredients, and cooking methods that mixed with local food cultures to make new recipes. Each American state is known for certain dishes, drinks, and snacks, depending on where each group of migrants settled. The best thing about these dishes is that they stand out from the original and if the Americans are right - they have been improved. Regardless of whether the French or the Belgians invented French fries, the Americans claim to have perfected it. Coleslaw, an indispensable side at any barbecue, is a slightly modified version of the "Koolsla" which comes from the Netherlands. Although apple pie came from England, it is now so American that it has its own expression: "as American as apple pie". It is always interesting to see how menu items change over time, how they are claimed by countries and cultures around the world. It is precisely this evolution of food and how people identify to them that continues even to this day. Adaptation to different economic circumstances, new technologies, and a variety of dietary restrictions guarantees it.

I have been living in the USA for a while now and belong to the category of '21st century immigrant'. I am contributing to the further development of these dishes too. When I started eating vegan several years ago, I felt like I was missing out on my favourite foods, especially barbecues. This feeling was short-lived as I was committed, despite my preferences, to enjoy traditional American food as much as any American. In addition, I had to give up gluten for health reasons and this posed yet another challenge for me. Always the adventurous type in the kitchen, I experimented with different recipes until I got the taste and texture of the food to be just as good as the original containing animal products and gluten.

I am a big fan of anything simple. That is why I like short ingredient lists and easy directions. Sometimes I use ready-to-use, gluten-free flour to simplify the task. If a list of ingredients is not too long, I "experiment" with flours and starches. During the development stages I noticed that, with many recipes, it does not matter what kind of plant-based milk you use, e.g. soy, almond, or cashew milk. In testing the dishes several times, I also noticed that, in some cases, it does not matter if you use refined, coconut, or brown sugar. So, if not specifically mentioned, when you read "sugar", it is up to you what kind to use. But if "brown sugar", for example, is explicitly listed, then use brown sugar. One thing is for sure, though, you do not have to live without your favourite American foods because of your lifestyle, and you can continue to feast in moderation the American way.

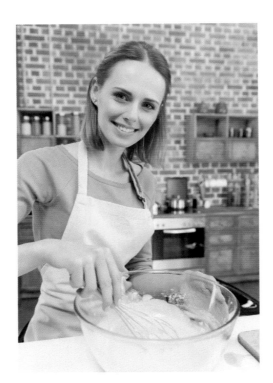

Now let us take you on a culinary journey through the USA. Enjoy every tasteful trip and make sure to share with friends and family; as Americans would say, the more the merrier!

Yours
Annette

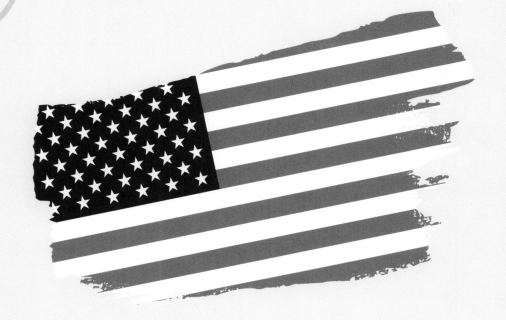

BREAKFAST

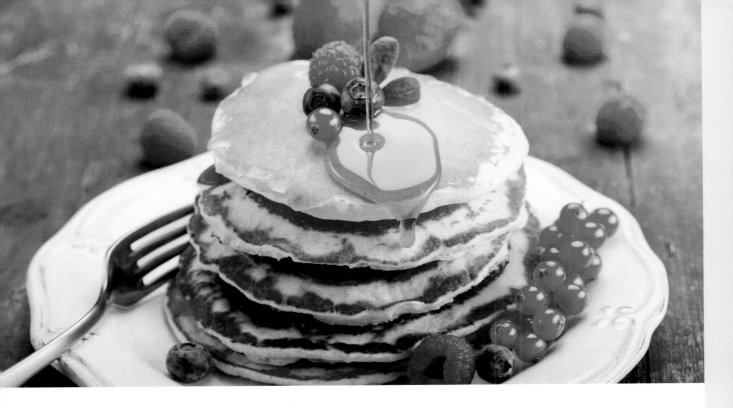

200g rice flour
60g tapioca flour (tapioca starch)
1 Tbsp linseed, ground
1 tsp baking powder
1/2 tsp salt
2 Tbsp of sugar
240 ml almond milk
60 ml oil
1 tsp apple cider vinegar

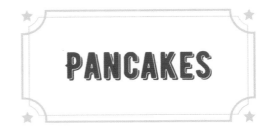

PANCAKES

Mix rice flour, tapioca, ground linseed, baking powder, salt and sugar in a bowl. Then add almond milk, oil, and apple cider vinegar and whisk.

Heat non-stick pan on medium heat. Pour dough in portions onto pan with small soup ladle or large spoon. The amount of dough depends on the preferred pancake size. As soon as the pancake forms bubbles, after 2-4 minutes, turn pancake over and cook for another 2 minutes or until golden brown before removing from heat. Repeat this process with the rest of the dough. Depending on the size of pancakes, quantity will be 6-9 pancakes. Serve with fruits, maple syrup, or icing sugar.

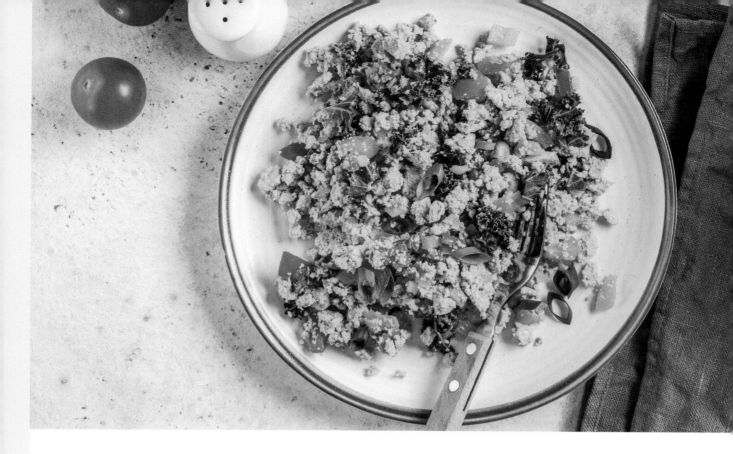

1-2 green onions, cut into thin strips
80g vegetables, diced (e.g. red peppers,
mushrooms, kale, tomatoes)
1/2 Tbsp oil
160g drained tofu, firm
1/4 tsp turmeric, ground
1/2 tsp nutritional yeast flakes
pinch of sweet paprika, ground
pinch of cayenne pepper, ground
Pinch of black salt (Kala Namak)
salt and black pepper, ground

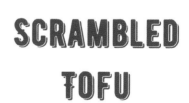

SCRAMBLED TOFU

Heat oil in pan and sauté onions until soft. Add diced vegetables and fry for a few minutes. Drain tofu, crumble finely with hands, then add to the pan. Add turmeric, nutritional yeast flakes, paprika, cayenne pepper, black salt, table salt and black pepper. Mix all ingredients well and stir-fry for a few minutes until the vegetables have softened and the tofu has acquired a yellow colour from the spices.

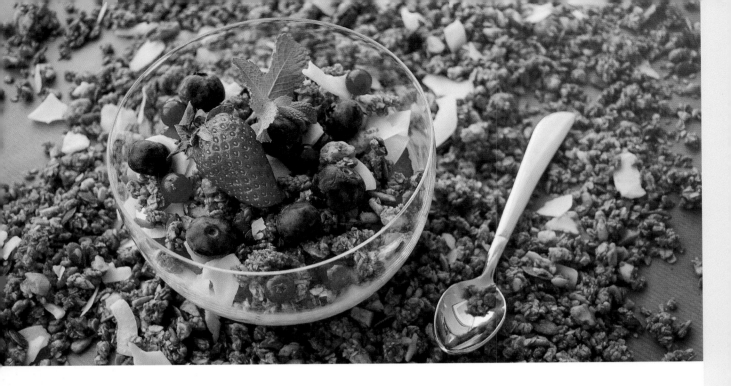

330g rolled oats, gluten-free
120g walnuts, chopped
3 Tbsp linseed, ground
2 tsp cinnamon, ground
1 tsp nutmeg, ground
1/2 tsp allspice, ground
1/2 tsp cloves, ground
1/2 tsp ginger, ground
1/4 tsp salt
80 ml maple syrup
60 ml apple juice or apple cider vinegar
1/2 tsp vanilla extract
Coconut chips (optional)

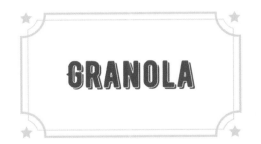

GRANOLA

Preheat oven to 160°C. Place oats, walnuts, ground linseed, cinnamon, nutmeg, allspice, cloves, ginger, and salt in a bowl and mix well. Add maple syrup, apple juice or vinegar, and vanilla extract and give it a good stir. Cover baking tray with baking paper and spread oat mixture evenly onto tray and bake for 25-30 minutes. Let cool and serve with fruits and plant-based milk. The granola can be stored in an airtight container. Also makes for great snacking.

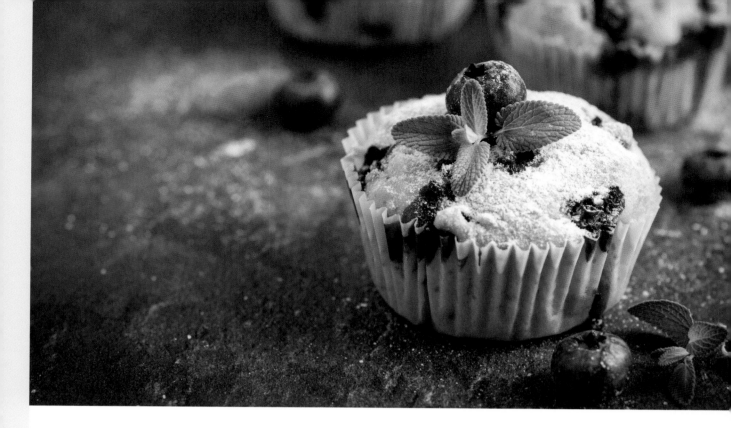

200g oat flour, gluten-free
40g rice flour
1 Tbsp linseed, ground
3 tsp baking powder
1/2 tsp salt
180 ml plant-based milk
120 ml maple syrup
80 ml oil
1 Tbsp apple cider vinegar
2 tsp vanilla extract
230g blueberries

BLUEBERRY MUFFINS

Preheat oven to 190°C. Put oat flour, rice flour, linseed, baking powder, and salt into bowl and mix well. Add plant-based milk, maple syrup, oil, apple cider vinegar, vanilla extract and stir well. Add blueberries and stir gently.
Grease muffin pan or line with muffin liners. Pour batter into pan and bake muffins for 20 minutes or until golden brown.
Sprinkle with icing sugar and serve. Makes 12 muffins.

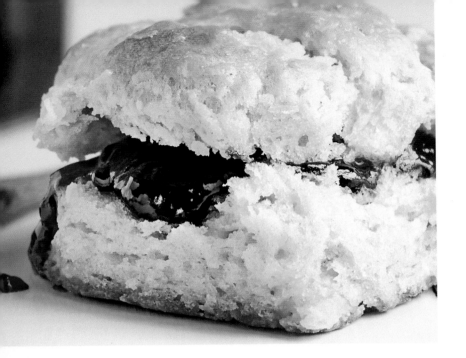

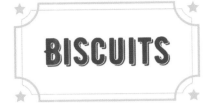

160g potato starch
10g corn starch
2 1/5 tsp baking powder
2 tsp nutritional yeast flakes
120 ml canned coconut milk

140g almond flour
1 tsp salt
12g sugar
60g vegan butter or margarine

Preheat oven to 200°C. Place potato starch, almond flour, corn starch, salt, baking powder, sugar, and nutritional yeast flakes in a bowl and mix well. Add vegan butter or margarine and work into the flour mix with a fork until consistent. While stirring, gradually add coconut milk until a sticky dough is formed. The dough should be neither too dry nor too wet. If necessary, add more coconut milk or more potato starch.

On a floured surface, flatten dough with floured hands until 2.5 – 3 cm thick. Cut out round or square shapes with floured cookie cutter or drinking glass. Place pieces on a baking tin lined with baking paper and brush with melted vegan butter or margarine.

Bake for 15 minutes, remove from oven and leave to cool for 10 minutes.

Serve warm with vegan butter or margarine and jam of your choice.

BANANA BREAD

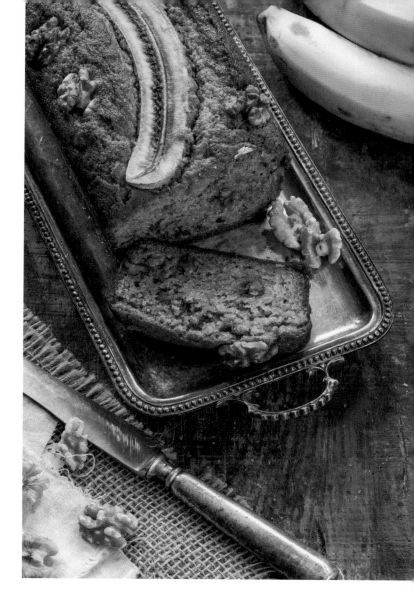

240g oat flour, gluten-free
1 tsp baking powder
1 tsp baking soda
1 tsp salt
1 tsp cinnamon, ground
1/2 tsp nutmeg, ground
4 ripe bananas
80 ml maple syrup
60 ml plant-based milk
60 ml oil
1 tsp vanilla extract
1 tsp apple cider vinegar
100g walnuts

Put oat flour, baking powder, baking soda, salt, and spices in a bowl and mix well.
Peel ripe bananas and in separate bowl either mash with a fork or purée in a mixer.
Add maple syrup, plant-based milk, oil, vanilla extract, and apple cider vinegar to the bananas and blend until smooth.
Add wet ingredients to the dry ingredients and mix well. Add 3/4 of the walnuts either whole or coarsely chopped to batter and stir.
Pour batter into a greased baking pan or casserole dish and sprinkle with the remaining walnuts. You can also decorate the batter with banana slices or half a banana.
Now place the dish in preheated oven and bake at 180°C for 55-60 minutes until the crust is golden brown. Let loaf cool and serve in slices.

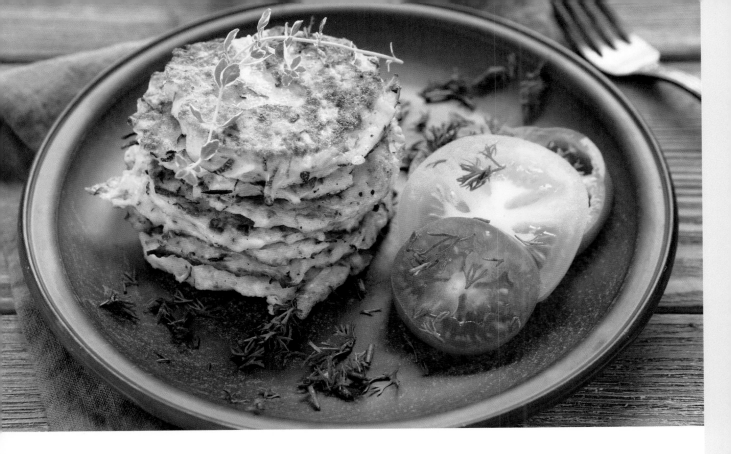

3 courgettes/zucchinis, medium-sized, grated
45g chickpea flour
3 green onions, cut into fine rings
1 Tbsp fresh parsley, chopped
1 Tbsp fresh dill, chopped
2 cloves of garlic, chopped
1 tsp salt
1/2 tsp oregano, dried
1/4 tsp black pepper, ground
oil for frying

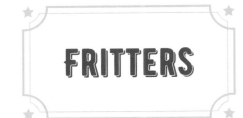

FRITTERS

Wring out grated courgettes/zucchinis and place in bowl. Add chickpea flour, green onions, parsley, dill, garlic, salt, oregano, and black pepper and mix well.
Heat oil in frying pan and add one heaping tablespoon of batter to form small flat cakes. Fry for 3-4 minutes each side until fritters are golden brown.
To remove excess oil, place fritters on a paper towel and serve warm. Makes about 12 fritters.

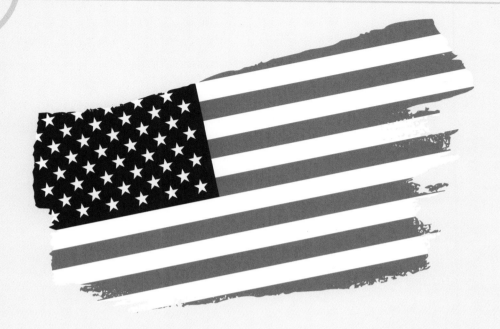

SOUPS

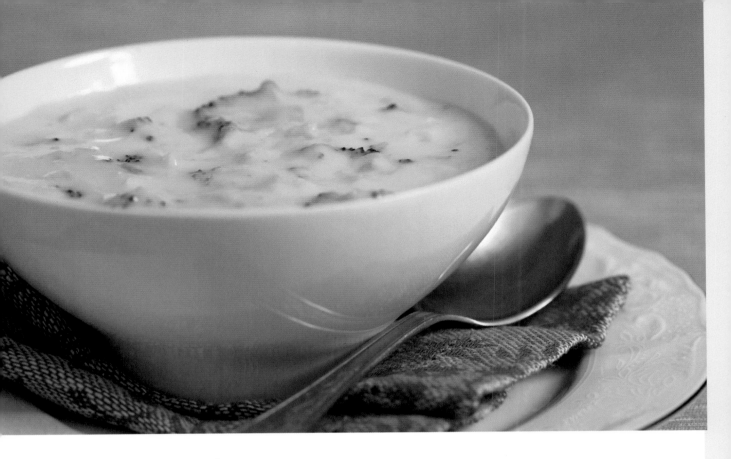

3 Tbsp oil
1/2 onion, large, finely chopped
30g rice flour
950 ml vegetable stock
240 ml water
2 Tbsp nutritional yeast flakes
900g fresh broccoli florets
60 ml almond milk
1/2 tsp salt
1/4 tsp black pepper, ground

CREAMY BROCCOLI SOUP

Heat oil in pot and sauté onion over medium heat until soft. Add rice flour, mix well and make a roux. While stirring constantly, gradually add broth, water, and nutritional yeast flakes and bring to a boil. Lower heat and simmer for 10 minutes, stirring frequently. Add broccoli and continue to cook for about 20 minutes, stirring occasionally, until the broccoli is soft. Add almond milk, salt, and black pepper. Purée lightly with a hand blender if desired. Makes 3-4 servings.

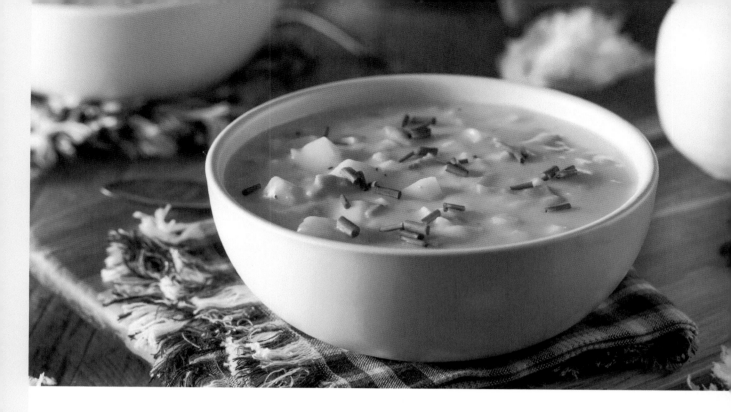

1 Tbsp oil
1/2 onion, large, diced
1 rib of celery, diced
1 red sweet pepper, diced
1 tin (~300 g) of sweetcorn
3 potatoes, peeled and diced
1/2 tsp thyme, dried
1/2 tsp oregano, dried
1/2 tsp salt
1/4 tsp black pepper, ground
30g rice flour
950 ml vegetable stock
240 ml plant-based milk

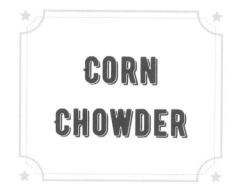

CORN CHOWDER

Heat oil in pot and sauté onion, celery and sweet peppers for 4-5 minutes. Drain corn and add it to pot, together with potatoes, thyme, oregano, salt, and pepper and mix well. Add rice flour and mix until the ingredients are evenly covered with flour. Add vegetable stock, stir and bring to a boil. Reduce heat and let simmer for about 20 minutes until the potatoes are soft. Add plant-based milk, stir and serve hot.

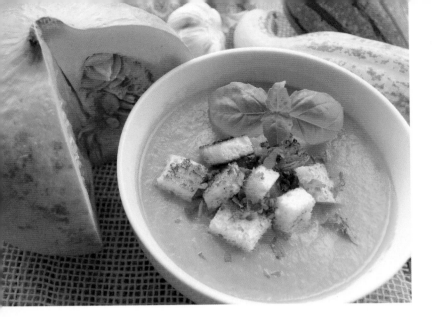

PUMPKIN SOUP WITH CROUTONS

red kuri squash or kabocha pumpkin (~450 g)
3 Tbsp oil
1 onion, large, chopped
1/2 tsp salt
1/2 tsp nutmeg, ground
1/8 tsp cayenne pepper, ground
1/4 tsp black pepper, ground
950 ml vegetable stock
120 ml canned coconut milk
2 Tbsp maple syrup

3 cloves of garlic, chopped
1/2 tsp cinnamon, ground
8 tsp cloves, ground

Croutons
2 slices of gluten-free bread (approx. 80 g)
1 Tbsp oil
1 garlic clove, pressed

Wash pumpkin or squash, quarter and remove seeds with spoon. Brush pumpkin/squash flesh with 1 Tbsp of oil and place it with flesh facing down on a baking tray lined with baking paper. Roast in preheated oven at 220°C for 35 minutes. Let it cool briefly, remove pumpkin/squash skin and cut flesh into small pieces.
In a pot heat 2 Tbsp of oil and sauté onion and garlic until soft. Add flesh pieces, salt, cinnamon, nutmeg, cloves, cayenne pepper, black pepper, and vegetable stock to the onion mixture and bring to a boil. Turn down heat and simmer for 15 minutes.
In the meantime, cut gluten-free bread slices into cubes. On low to medium heat, heat 1 Tbsp of oil in frying pan and fry the pressed garlic and bread cubes for about 5 minutes, turning the bread cubes regularly.
Now add the coconut milk and maple syrup to the soup and purée with a hand blender. Serve the soup with croutons.

18

ROASTED CAULIFLOWER SOUP

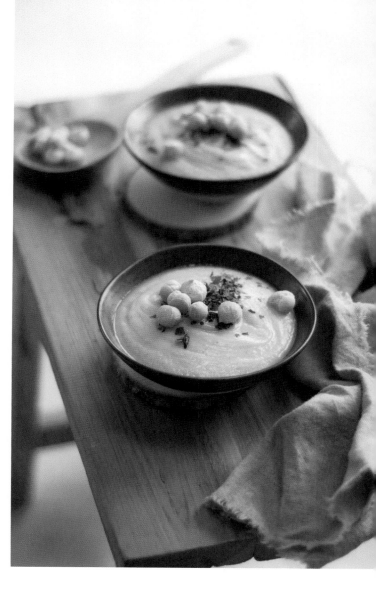

1 head of cauliflower, medium-sized
2 Tbsp oil
1/4 tsp cumin, ground
1 tsp salt
200g chickpeas, canned
1/4 tsp chipotle powder / chili powder
1/2 onion, large, diced
1 clove of garlic, chopped
950 ml vegetable stock
1/4 tsp black pepper, ground
2 Tbsp parsley, dried

Remove leaves and stalk from cauliflower. Quarter the head and cut off stalk from each quarter so that the florets fall off. Break large florets apart with your hands and give them a rinse.
In a bowl, mix the small florets with 1/2 Tbsp of oil, cumin, and 1/2 tsp of salt and place on a baking tray lined with baking paper. Drain chickpeas and put into the mixing bowl, add 1/2 Tbsp of oil and chipotle powder. Put chickpeas on baking tray next to florets. Roast in a preheated oven at 200°C for 20 minutes.
In a pot heat 1 Tbsp of oil and sauté onion and garlic until soft. Add roasted florets and vegetable stock. Purée with a hand blender. Add 1/2 tsp salt and 1/4 tsp black pepper. Bring to a boil while stirring. Serve with the roasted chickpeas and dried parsley.

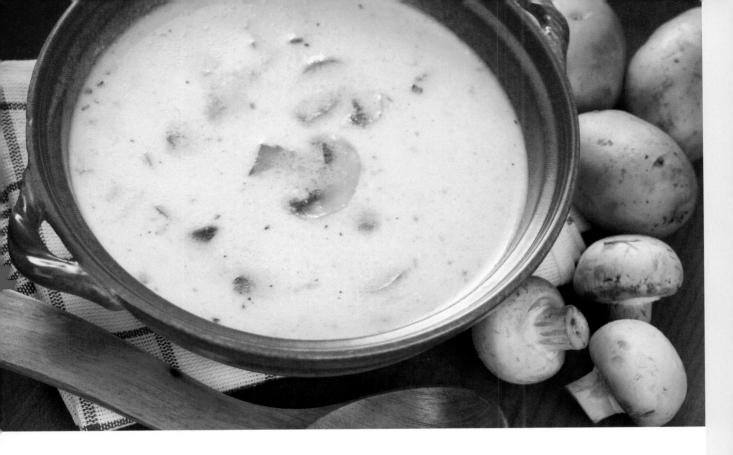

2 Tbsp oil
1/2 onion, large, finely chopped
230g fresh mushrooms, sliced
2 cloves of garlic, chopped
30g rice flour
1/2 tsp salt
1/4 tsp black pepper, ground
1/4 tsp nutmeg, ground
1/4 tsp thyme, dried
950 ml vegetable stock
240 ml plant-based milk

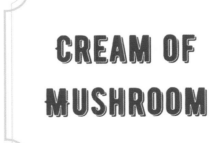

CREAM OF MUSHROOM

Heat oil in pot and sauté onion and mushrooms at medium heat for 3-4 minutes. Add garlic and sauté for another minute. Then add rice flour, salt, black pepper, nutmeg, and thyme and mix well. Pour in vegetable stock and plant-based milk, stir well and bring to a boil. Reduce heat and let simmer for 15-20 minutes, stirring frequently, until soup has thickened. Serve hot. Serves 4-5.

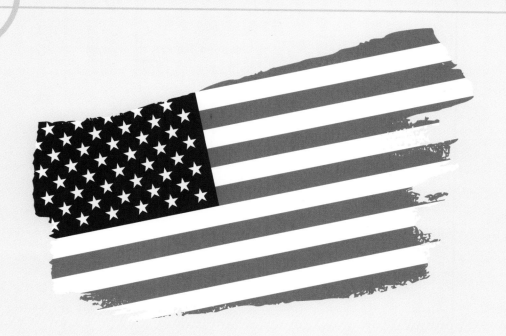

MAINS

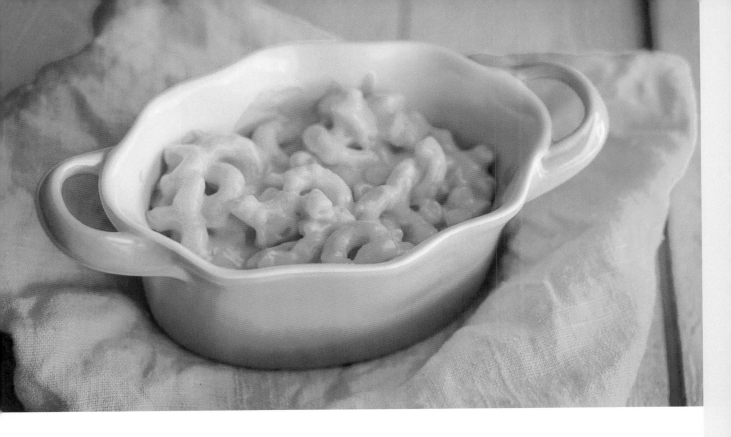

250g macaroni pasta, gluten-free

Sauce
2 potatoes, medium-sized, peeled and diced
1 carrot, medium-sized, diced
4 Tbsp nutritional yeast flakes
120 ml cooking water
1 tsp apple cider vinegar
1/2 tsp garlic powder
1 tsp salt

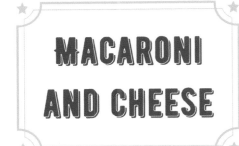

MACARONI AND CHEESE

Cook macaroni pasta according to the package instructions.
In a pot bring water to a boil and cook the carrot and potatoes over medium heat until soft. Put 120 ml of the cooking water into a blender or food processor. Add the drained vegetables, nutritional yeast flakes, vinegar, garlic powder, and salt to the blender and blend the sauce ingredients into a creamy mixture on high to medium speed for 1-2 minutes.
Cover prepared macaroni with the sauce, stir well and serve warm.

SHEPHERD'S PIE

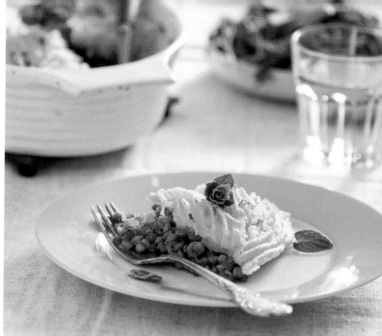

Vegetable Filling
2 Tbsp oil
1 onion, medium-sized, diced
2 cloves of garlic, chopped
150g carrots, diced
150g green lentils, cooked, e.g. from a tin
75g peas
75g sweetcorn, canned
2 Tbsp rice flour
1 Tbsp thyme, dried
1 tsp salt
1/2 tsp black pepper, ground
120 ml vegetable stock

Mashed Potatoes
1,5 L water
salt
900g potatoes, peeled and diced
1 Tbsp vegan margarine
1 Tbsp plant-based milk
black pepper, ground

For the mashed potatoes: In a pot bring water to a boil, add salt and diced potatoes and let simmer at medium heat until potatoes are soft. Meanwhile heat oil in another pot to prepare vegetable filling. Add onion, garlic, and carrots and sauté until soft for a few minutes. Add lentils, peas, and corn and sauté for a few minutes more. Cover vegetables with rice flour, thyme, salt, and pepper and mix well. Add vegetable stock and bring to a boil while stirring until the vegetable mixture has thickened. Drain potatoes and add vegan margarine, plant-based milk, salt, and pepper as desired while mashing. Put vegetable mixture into a greased casserole dish and spread the mashed potatoes evenly over vegetable mixture. Bake in a preheated oven at 200°C for 25 minutes until potato crust begins to brown. Serve with fresh herbs as desired.

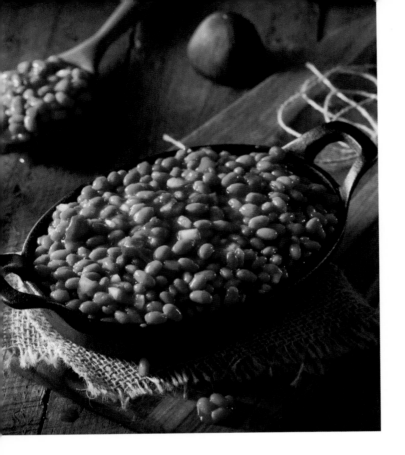

BARBECUE BAKED BEANS

300g small white beans, dry OR 500-600g drained white beans from a can

1 Tbsp oil

1 onion, large, chopped

1 sweet pepper, red, diced

60 ml apple cider vinegar

1 Tbsp of mustard

1 bay leaf

1/2 tsp chili powder or chili flakes

1 tsp black pepper, ground

240 ml water

3 cloves of garlic, chopped

800g chopped tomatoes from a can

3 Tbsp blackstrap molasses

1 tsp cumin, ground

1 tsp rosemary, dried

2 tsp salt

1 Tbsp smoked paprika, ground

When using dry beans, soak the beans in water overnight and drain. Put fresh water in a pot and cook beans for 60-90 minutes until soft, then drain and put aside. Heat oil in a pot and sauté onion and garlic for a few minutes. Add diced sweet pepper and sauté until soft. Now add beans along with all remaining ingredients, mix well and cook covered on low to medium heat for about 40-60 minutes, until thickened. Serves 4-6.

STUFFED PEPPERS

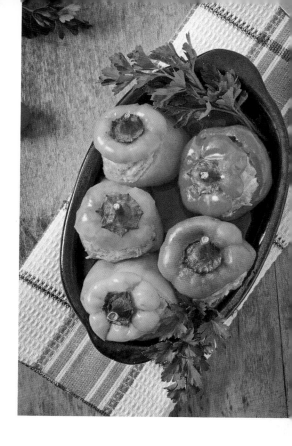

150g brown rice
4-5 sweet peppers, red, orange, yellow and green
1 Tbsp oil
1 onion, medium-sized, diced
2 cloves of garlic, chopped
1 rib of celery, diced
100g tomatoes, fresh, diced or chopped from a can
1 Tbsp tomato paste
1/2 tsp salt
1/2 tsp sage, dried
1/4 tsp garlic powder
handful breadcrumbs, gluten-free (optional)
2-3 Tbsp water

1/4 tsp basil, dried
1/4 tsp thyme, dried
15g walnuts, chopped
handful grated vegan cheese

Cook rice according to package instructions and put aside. Wash sweet peppers and cut off the "lid" (see photo). Remove seeds.
Heat oil in frying pan and sauté onion, garlic cloves, and celery until soft. Add tomatoes and tomato paste and sauté for a few more minutes. Add salt and remaining spices and mix well. Combine mixture with chopped walnuts, cooked rice and, if desired, gluten-free breadcrumbs and mix well. Fill peppers with mixture.
Place stuffed peppers upright in a roaster or high casserole dish. Sprinkle with vegan grated cheese and place the pepper lids on top. If there is any filling left over due to the different sizes and number of peppers, dilute it with water and add it to the roaster or casserole dish. Cover the dish with a lid or aluminium foil and bake in a preheated oven at 180°C for 45 minutes. Then remove the aluminium foil and bake for another 10 minutes. Serve hot.

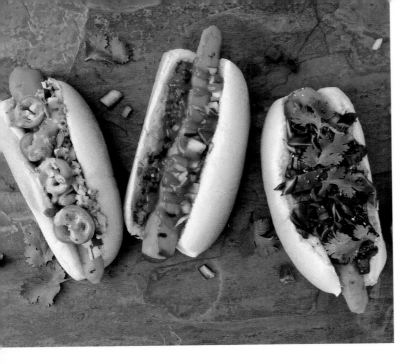

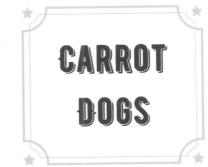

CARROT DOGS

4 carrots, large   water

Marinade

125 ml tamari sauce   125 ml apple cider vinegar   125 ml water
2 Tbsp maple syrup   2 tsp sweet paprika, ground   2 tsp garlic powder
1/2 tsp black pepper, ground

4 gluten-free, vegan hot dog buns

Peel and wash carrots and shorten them to the size of the hot dog buns if desired. Bring a pot of water to a boil and simmer the carrots for 20-30 minutes on medium heat.

In the meantime, prepare the marinade. Pour tamari sauce, apple cider vinegar, water, maple syrup, and spices into a flat storage container and mix well. Drain carrots and place them in marinade container. Roll them so that they are well covered with the marinade. Close the container and store in the refrigerator for 24 hours.

The next day, remove the carrots. Do not throw the marinade out, it can be used in a stir-fry, for example. Fry the carrots on a contact grill or in a pan for 5-10 minutes. Then place them in gluten-free vegan hot dog buns and dress with ketchup, mustard, and toppings like roasted or fresh onions, tomatoes, sweet pepper or cabbage. Enjoy!

BARBECUE TOFU

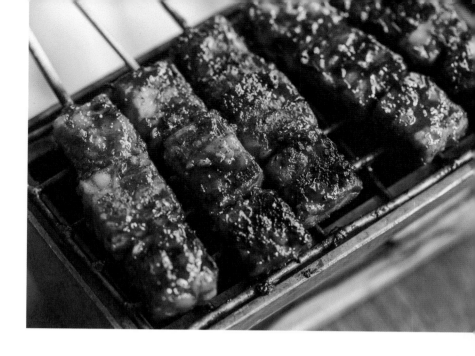

Sauce

170g tomato paste
1 Tbsp pomegranate syrup
1 Tbsp tamari sauce
1/2 Tbsp onion powder
1 tsp salt
60 ml water

180 ml apple cider vinegar
4 Tbsp maple syrup
1/2 Tbsp garlic powder
1 1/2 tsp sweet paprika, ground
1 tsp black pepper, ground

400g tofu, firm, drained and cut into cubes
oil for the pan

Place tomato paste, vinegar, pomegranate syrup, maple syrup, tamari sauce, garlic powder, onion powder, paprika, salt, pepper, and water in a saucepan and whisk well until smooth. Let the sauce thicken for 10-15 minutes over low to medium heat, stirring constantly. Remove from heat and set aside.
Either skewer the tofu pieces and put them on the grill or heat some oil in a grill pan and fry the tofu pieces on all sides over medium to high heat until grill stripes appear on the tofu. Brush the tofu pieces with the barbecue sauce on all sides and place them on the grill or grill pan for another minute. Brush the pieces with the sauce again and grill them again. Repeat this process 2-3 times. If there is any barbecue sauce left, use it for stir-fry dishes or as a marinade.

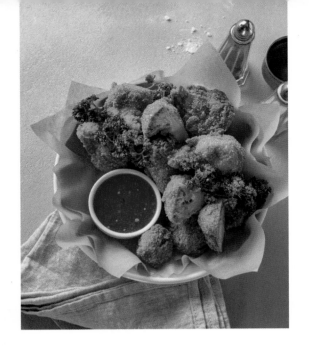

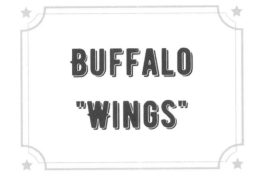

BUFFALO "WINGS"

1 head cauliflower (or broccoli)

Coating
250 ml plant-based milk
120g chickpea flour
1 tsp. onion powder
1 tsp garlic powder
1/2 tsp salt
1/4 tsp sweet paprika, ground
1/8 tsp black pepper, ground

Buffalo Sauce
125 ml water
4 Tbsp apple cider vinegar
4 Tbsp tomato paste
2 Tbsp tamari sauce
2 Tbsp tahini (sesame paste)
2 tsp sweet paprika, ground
2 tsp garlic powder
1/2 tsp cayenne pepper, ground

Remove leaves and stalk from cauliflower. Quarter the head and cut off the stalk on each quarter so that the florets fall off. Break up large florets with your hands into bite-size pieces.

In a bowl, mix well all ingredients for the coating until there are no more lumps. Put the florets into the bowl and toss until all florets are well covered.

Place the florets on a baking tray covered with baking paper and bake in a preheated oven at 230°C for 20 minutes, turning once halfway through cooking time.

Place all ingredients for the buffalo sauce in a bowl and stir until smooth. Dip the florets in the sauce, shake off excess sauce and place the florets back on the baking tray. Bake the florets for another 20 minutes until they are golden brown, turning them at halfway. For extra spiciness, serve the "wings" with chilli sauce.

NEATLOAF

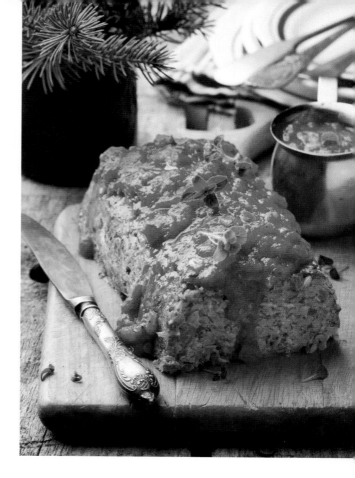

200g millet
700 ml vegetable stock
3 potatoes, peeled and diced
3 Tbsp oil
3 onions, small, chopped
3 cloves of garlic, chopped
2 ribs of celery, diced
1 tsp cumin, ground
1 tsp sage, dried
1 tsp thyme, dried
1 tsp salt
2 Tbsp balsamic vinegar

Sauce

150g canned tomatoes, chopped   2 Tbsp mustard   2 Tbsp brown sugar
2 Tbsp vinegar

Wash millet by putting in a fine mesh colander and rinsing under running water. In a saucepan bring vegetable stock to a boil, add millet and cook for about 20 minutes on low heat until the millet has absorbed most of the liquid. Allow to cool.

Wash, peel and dice potatoes and cook them in a separate pot until soft. Drain and cool.

Heat oil in a pan and sauté onions and garlic cloves for a few minutes. Add celery and sauté until everything is soft. Add cumin, sage, thyme, and salt, turn down heat completely and deglaze the onion mixture with balsamic vinegar and let it cool down. Place the cooled millet, potatoes, and onion mixture in a mixing bowl and knead well with your hands. Line a bread baking form with baking paper, press the mixture into the form and bake in a preheated oven at 180°C for 30-45 minutes.

Mix the tomato sauce ingredients in a bowl. After loaf has cooled a bit, cut into slices and serve with sauce. Serves 4-6 people.

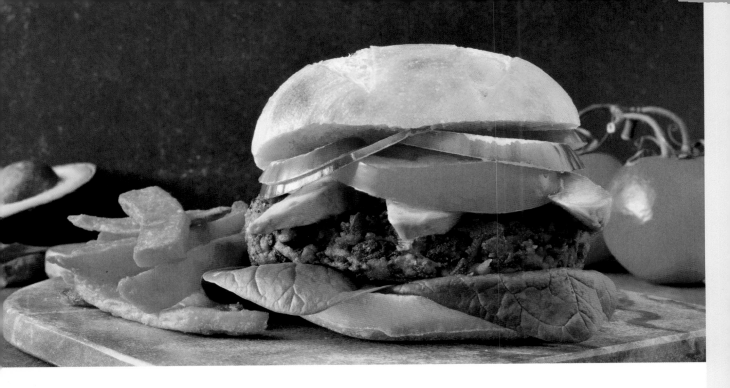

1 Tbsp chia seeds + 3 Tbsp water
1/2 sweet pepper, green, chopped
1/2 onion, medium-sized, chopped
2 cloves of garlic, chopped
handful fresh coriander leaves
1 Tbsp chili powder
1 Tbsp cumin, ground
1 tsp sweet paprika, ground
1 tsp salt
240g black beans from the tin
65g rolled oats, gluten-free

BLACK BEAN BURGER PATTIES

Mix chia seeds and water and set aside for 15 minutes.
Put coarsely chopped pepper and onion, cloves of garlic, coriander leaves, and spices in a food processor and chop finely. Add chia seeds, well drained canned black beans, and oats to the chopped vegetables and turn the food processor on briefly until everything is well combined. Let the mixture rest in the refrigerator for one hour, then form 4 patties of the same size and place them on a baking tray with baking paper. Bake in a preheated oven at 190°C for 10 minutes. Turn patties and bake another 10 minutes. Serve with gluten-free hamburger buns and preferred toppings such as sauces, lettuce or spinach, avocado, tomatoes, and onion.

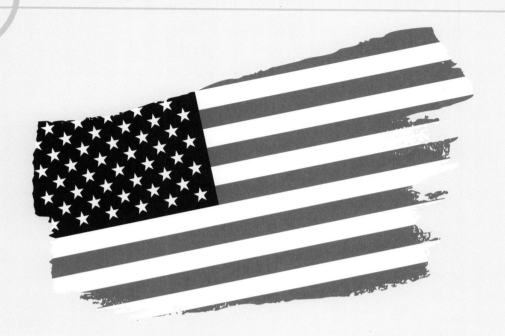

SIDES

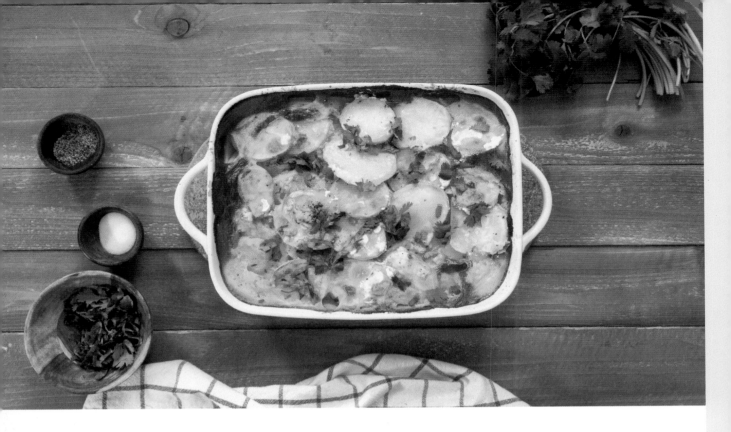

1 kg potatoes, thinly sliced
3 Tbsp oil
1 onion, small, chopped
1 garlic clove, chopped
2 Tbsp rice flour
2 Tbsp nutritional yeast flakes
1 tsp salt
1/4 tsp black pepper, ground
550 ml almond milk

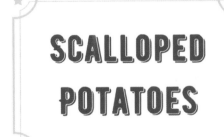

SCALLOPED POTATOES

Wash and peel potatoes and cut into thin slices.

Heat oil in a pot and sauté chopped onion and garlic for a few minutes. Add rice flour, nutritional yeast flakes, salt, and pepper and make a roux. Slowly add the almond milk, stirring constantly to avoid lumps. Bring to a boil while stirring until the sauce thickens.

Grease an oven dish, place potatoes in it and cover evenly with the sauce. Cover the casserole dish with aluminium foil and bake in preheated oven at 180°C for 30 minutes. Remove the foil and continue baking for about 20 minutes.

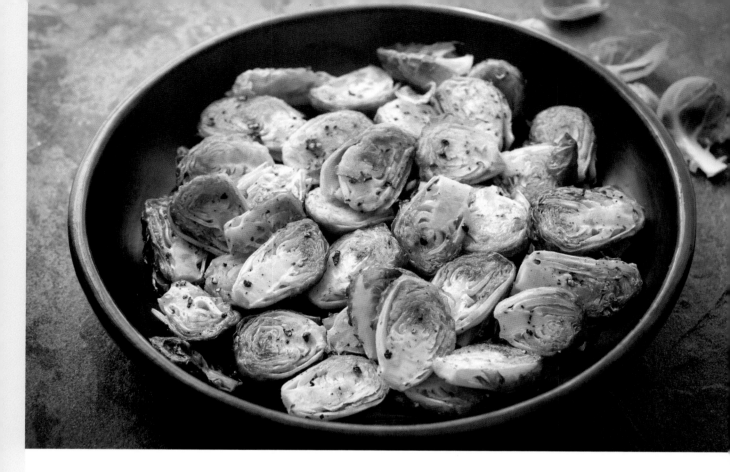

1 kg brussels sprouts
salt
black pepper, ground
1 tsp rosemary, dried
3 Tbsp oil
1/2 Tbsp balsamic vinegar

ROASTED BRUSSEL SPROUTS

Remove yellowed leaves and stalks from brussels sprouts. Wash brussels sprouts, dry well and cut in halves. Place the sprouts in a mixing bowl. Mix with salt, pepper, rosemary, oil, and vinegar and then spread on a baking tray covered with baking paper. Place the sprouts with the cut surface facing up. Bake in a preheated oven at 200°C for 15 minutes. Then turn the brussels sprouts and bake for another 10 minutes.

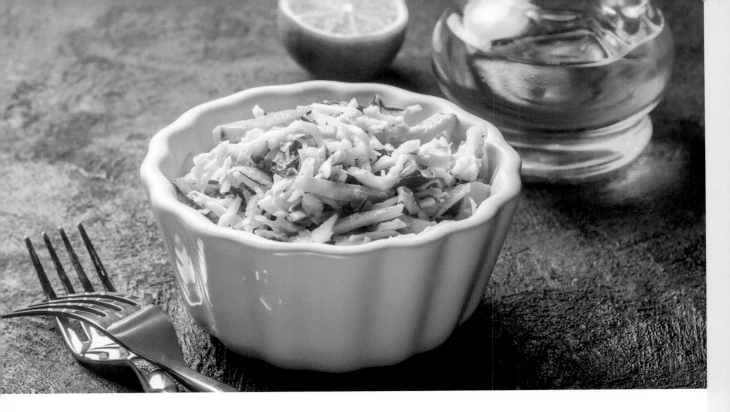

300g white cabbage, cut into fine strips
100g red cabbage, cut into fine strips
1 onion, medium-sized, cut into fine strips
1 carrot, large, grated or cut into fine strips

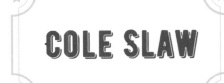

COLE SLAW

<u>Dressing</u>

3 Tbsp apple cider vinegar 3 Tbsp oil
1/2 Tbsp mustard 1 tsp celery seed
1 Tbsp maple syrup 1/4 tsp salt
1/4 tsp black pepper, ground

If you like it creamy, add 200g of vegan and gluten-free mayonnaise.

Put cut white cabbage, red cabbage, onion, and carrot into a large bowl and mix well. Whisk apple cider vinegar, oil, mustard, celery seed, maple syrup, salt, and pepper (and for the creamy version, mayonnaise) together in a small bowl and pour over the cabbage blend. Mix well until the cabbage is completely covered.
Chill in refrigerator for a few hours before serving.

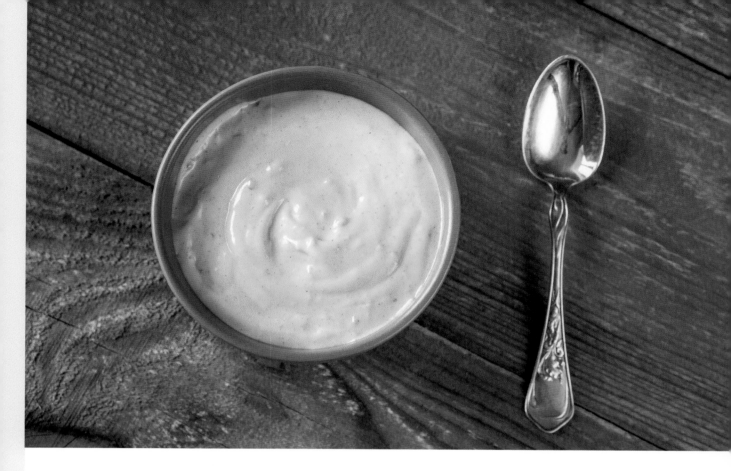

75g cashews, unsalted
120 ml water
60 ml lemon juice
450g tofu, firm
1/2 tsp salt
1 tsp onion powder
2 tsp maple syrup
225g tomato purée
1 tsp garlic powder

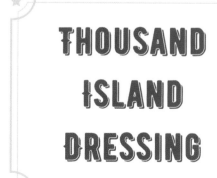

THOUSAND ISLAND DRESSING

Soak cashews in water for 6 hours, drain and put them together with all the other ingredients into a food processor or blender and blend until smooth.
Chill in refrigerator for an hour before serving.
Goes well with salads, is suitable as a dip or can be used as a burger sauce.

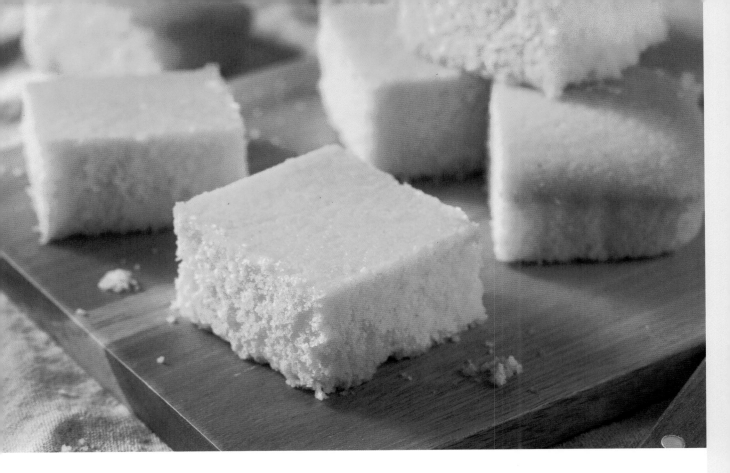

240 ml almond milk
3 Tbsp oil
1/2 tsp apple cider vinegar
230g corn flour
120g oat flour, gluten-free
60g sugar
1 Tbsp baking powder
1/2 tsp salt

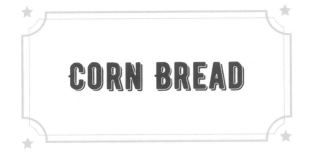

CORN BREAD

Put almond milk, oil, and apple cider vinegar in a bowl and mix well. Add corn flour, oat flour, sugar, baking powder, and salt. Mix to form a batter.
Pour batter into a greased baking dish and distribute evenly.
Bake in a preheated oven at 200°C for 20-25 minutes. Let cool, cut into squares and serve with beans or soups.

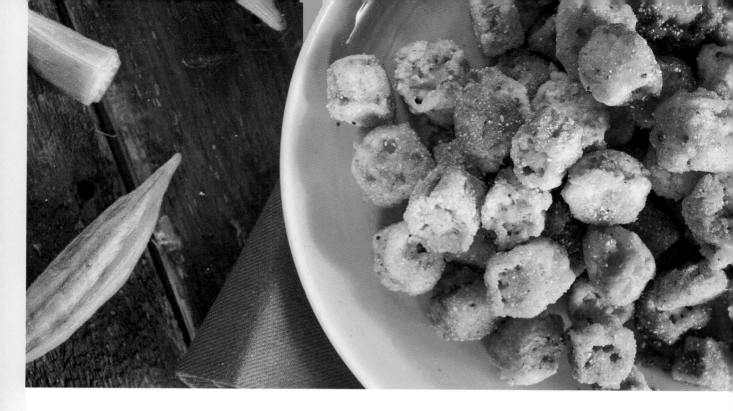

200g fresh okra pods
80 ml almond milk
1 tsp vinegar
50g rice flour
50g corn flour
10g nutritional yeast flakes
1 tsp salt
1/4 tsp black pepper, ground
1/4 tsp garlic powder
pinch of cayenne pepper, ground

OVEN FRIED OKRA

Wash okra pods, discard the ends and cut the okra into 1 cm thick slices. Mix almond milk and vinegar and put aside. Put rice flour, corn flour, nutritional yeast flakes, salt, pepper, garlic powder, and cayenne pepper in a bowl and mix well.
Dip the slices of okra into the almond milk mixture first and then toss them in the flour mixture so that the slices are evenly coated on all sides. Then spread the slices on a baking tray covered with baking paper and bake in a preheated oven at 230°C for 10-12 minutes. Turn okra slices and bake for another 10-12 minutes and serve immediately.

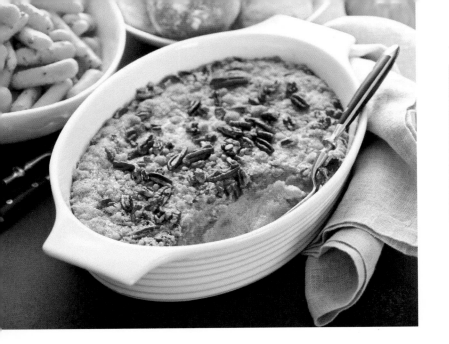

SWEET POTATO CASSEROLE

4 sweet potatoes, medium-sized
water
pinch of salt
2 Tbsp vegan margarine
60 ml maple syrup
60 ml almond milk, unsweetened
3 Tbsp coconut sugar or brown sugar
pinch of cinnamon, ground

Topping
100g pecans
40g rice flour
60g coconut sugar or brown sugar
4 Tbsp oil
pinch of salt

Wash, peel and dice sweet potatoes. Bring water to a boil in a saucepan, add potatoes and a pinch of salt and cook for about 15 minutes at medium heat until soft.

In the meantime, put topping ingredients in a food processor or blender and blend to a chunky composition.

Place drained potatoes in bowl, add 2 Tbsp of vegan margarine and mash potatoes. Add maple syrup, almond milk, sugar, a pinch of salt, and cinnamon and mix to a smooth and creamy texture. Use a food processor or a blender if needed.

Spread sweet potato mixture evenly into an oven dish. Pour topping mixture over it and cover potatoes completely. If desired, top with a handful of very roughly chopped pecans.

Bake in a preheated oven at 190°C for 30-35 minutes until crust is golden brown.

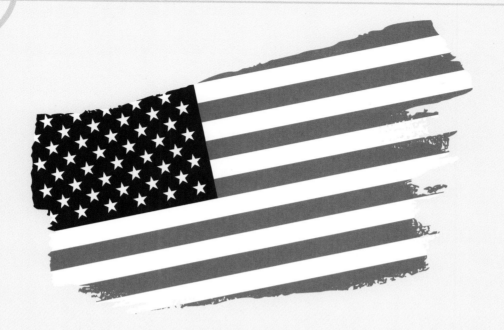

DESSERTS

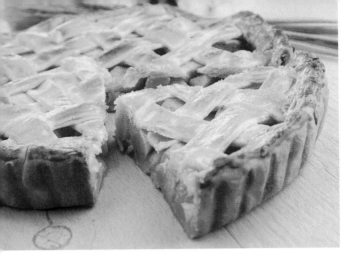

APPLE PIE

Crust
90g oat flour, gluten-free
160g rice flour
1 Tbsp tapioca flour/starch
1/2 tsp salt
150g vegan margarine
2-3 Tbsp water

Filling
6-7 apples
65g sugar
3 Tbsp rice flour
1 tsp cinnamon, ground
1/2 tsp nutmeg, ground
1/4 tsp vanilla extract
1/8 tsp salt
1 Tbsp vegan margarine

Glaze
2 Tbsp almond milk   1 tsp agave syrup

Put oat flour, rice flour, tapioca, and salt in a bowl and mix well. Add vegan margarine and work it evenly into the mixture. Add one Tbsp of water at a time and knead the dough well with your hands to get a nice ball of dough. Cut dough in half, wrap both parts in cling film/plastic wrap and place in the fridge for 15 minutes.

Peel apples, cut into thin slices and put in a bowl. Sprinkle apples with sugar, rice flour, cinnamon, nutmeg, vanilla extract, and salt and mix until the apples are well covered with the sugar mixture.

Place one half of the dough on baking paper and roll out to a 23 cm diameter circle. Carefully lift and flip the baking paper and dough into a pie dish. Peel baking paper off dough. Align the dough edges with pie dish edges.

To make the grid pattern (see photo), roll out the other half of the dough and cut it into strips of varying lengths upto 23 cm, each one 2 cm wide.

Put the apple mixture into the pie dish and distribute evenly. Divide 1 Tbsp margarine into small pieces and place on the apples.

Now lay the dough strips on the apples and create a grid pattern. Press down the edges of the dough with your fingers. Mix the almond milk and agave syrup and brush it onto the grid form. Bake in preheated oven at 190°C for 45 minutes and let cool before cutting.

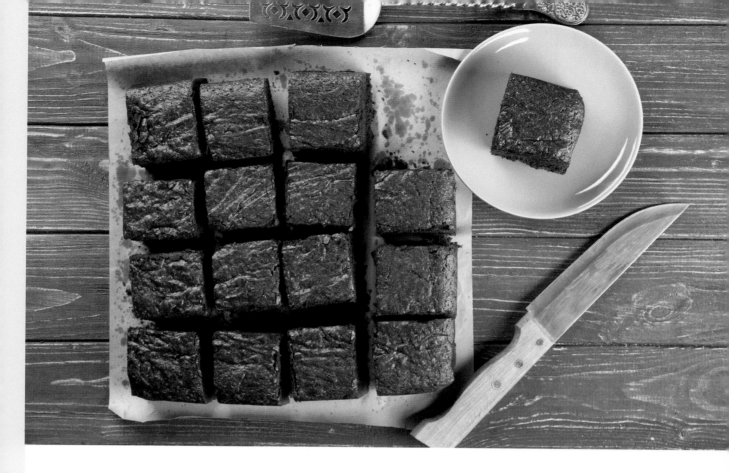

2 Tbsp linseed, ground	6 Tbsp water
60g almond butter	80g sugar
60 ml maple syrup	70 ml oil
75g unsweetened cocoa powder	1 tsp vanilla extract
1/4 tsp salt	40g oat flour
90g vegan chocolate chips	oil for the baking tray

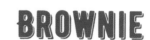

BROWNIE

Mix linseed and water and put aside for 15 minutes.

Put almond butter, sugar, maple syrup, and oil in a bowl and mix well with a whisk until a caramel-like batter is formed. Gradually add cocoa powder while stirring. Also add vanilla extract and salt. Now stir in the soaked linseed. Slowly add the flour until you have a smooth, firm batter. Mix in the chocolate chips and place the dough in a greased square metal tray (20 x 20 cm) lined with baking paper. Bake in a preheated oven at 160°C for 30-35 minutes. Perform a toothpick test. Properly cooked dough should not stick to the toothpick. Allow to cool completely before cutting into squares. Makes 16 brownies.

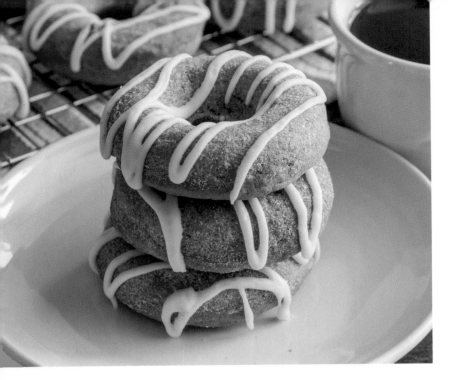

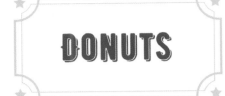

DONUTS

Dough
200g gluten-free flour
120 ml almond milk
4 Tbsp maple syrup
2 Tbsp coconut oil, melted
1/4 tsp vanilla extract
oil for the doughnut baking tin

Cinnamon Sugar
5 Tbsp sugar
1 tsp cinnamon, ground

Glaze
2 Tbsp almond milk
140g icing sugar, sieved

Place gluten-free flour, almond milk, maple syrup, coconut oil, and vanilla extract in a bowl and combine to a smooth batter.

Grease a 6-cavity doughnut baking tin with vegan margarine or coconut oil and fill the dough into the baking tin. Bake in a preheated oven at 180°C for about 14 minutes. If necessary, perform a toothpick test.

Meanwhile, put the cinnamon and sugar in a bowl and mix well.

Allow the donuts to cool for 5 minutes and then take them out of the baking tin. A toothpick can help get them out easily.

Dip the still hot and greased side of the donuts into the cinnamon sugar and let it cool on a grid.

Then mix sifted icing sugar and almond milk and pour over the donuts.

FUDGE

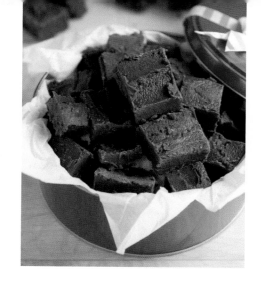

90g vegan chocolate, chopped or chips
120g almond butter or tahini (sesame paste)
1/2 tsp peppermint extract or vanilla extract

Water bath: Heat water in a large pot and place a small pot in it. Chop the chocolate if necessary, put into small pot and let the chocolate melt while stirring. Add almond butter or tahini and the extract and mix well.
Pour the mixture into a small tin or casserole dish lined with baking paper, spread evenly and smooth it down. Place the dish in the freezer for 40 minutes and then cut into small squares.

PEANUT BUTTER COOKIES

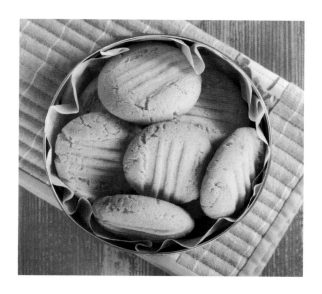

150g peanut butter
50g sugar
75 ml plant-based milk
75g oat flour, gluten-free
chocolate chips (optional)

Put peanut butter, sugar, plant-based milk, and oat flour in a bowl, mix well and form a dough. Make 12 biscuits and place them on a baking tray covered with baking paper. Create lines on the biscuits with a fork and if desired, add vegan chocolate chips onto the biscuits. Bake in a preheated oven at 180°C for 10 minutes.

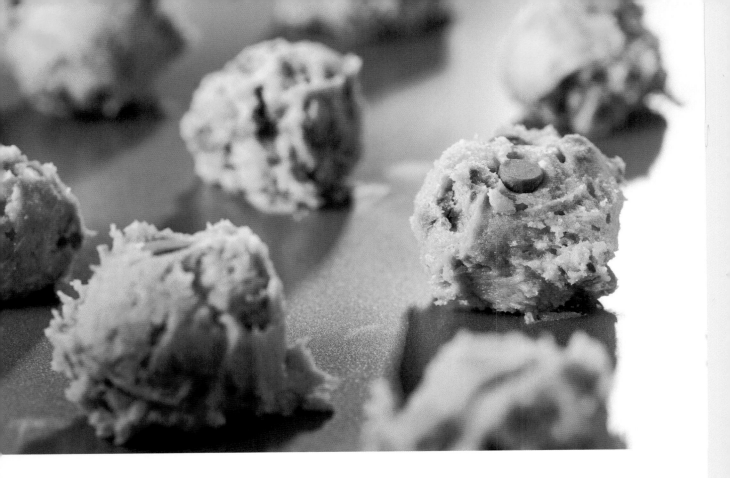

100g almond flour
30g oat flour, gluten-free
75 ml maple syrup
1 Tbsp coconut oil, melted
2 Tbsp almond milk
1/2 tsp vanilla extract
1/2 tsp salt
45g vegan chocolate chips

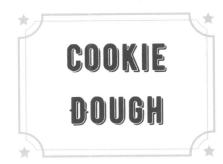

COOKIE DOUGH

Place all ingredients in a bowl, mix well and form a dough. Make small balls and place them in the freezer for 15 minutes. Serve with ice cream or just eat it as is (raw).

Alternatively, the dough balls can be baked in a preheated oven at 180°C for 10 minutes and consumed like "real" biscuits/cookies.

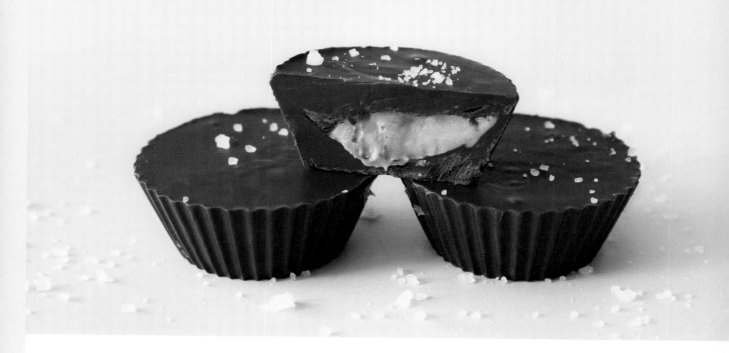

240g vegan chocolate, chopped or chips
60g peanut butter
1 Tbsp maple syrup
1/4 tsp salt, coarse

PEANUT BUTTER CUPS

Water bath: Heat water in a small pot and place a bowl over it. Chop the chocolate if necessary, put into the bowl and let the chocolate melt while stirring.
In a separate bowl mix peanut butter and maple syrup.
Into each of 8 muffin moulds (silicone or paper) put one Tbsp of melted chocolate.
Place muffin moulds in freezer for 10 minutes to allow the chocolate to set.
Then place 1-2 tsp of peanut butter mix on the chocolate in each mould and press flat.
Spread the rest of the melted chocolate on the muffin moulds, smooth it down, sprinkle with coarse-grained salt and place in the freezer for 15 minutes until the top layer of chocolate is also firm.
Place in an airtight container at room temperature so that the cups are not too hard when you bite into them.

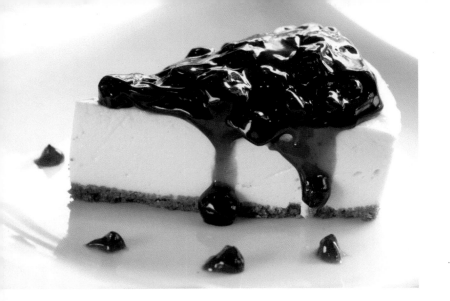

CHEESE CAKE

Crust
melted coconut oil for springform
40g walnuts
40g almonds
100g dates, pitted
pinch of salt

Filling
200g cashews, unsalted
180g coconut cream, solid part from a can of coconut milk
30 ml maple syrup
40g coconut oil, melted
2 Tbsp lemon juice
1/4 tsp vanilla extract

Sauce
150g blueberries, fresh or frozen
2 Tbsp maple syrup

For the filling: soak cashews in water for 6 hours.

Line a springform pan (18 cm or 22 cm – the bigger the springform pan, the flatter the cake) with baking paper and brush the sides with melted coconut oil.

Put remaining ingredients for the crust into a food processor, chop it up and make a sticky mixture. Press the mixture into the springform pan evenly. Place the springform pan in the freezer for a few minutes.

Drain the cashews and put them in the food processor with the remaining ingredients for the filling and create a smooth cream. Pour the cream onto the cake crust and this time put it in the freezer for about 1 hour.

In the meantime, place the blueberries and maple syrup in a saucepan and cook over low heat, stirring regularly, for 10 minutes and then leave to cool. When serving, pour the sauce over the cake.

PEACH COBBLER

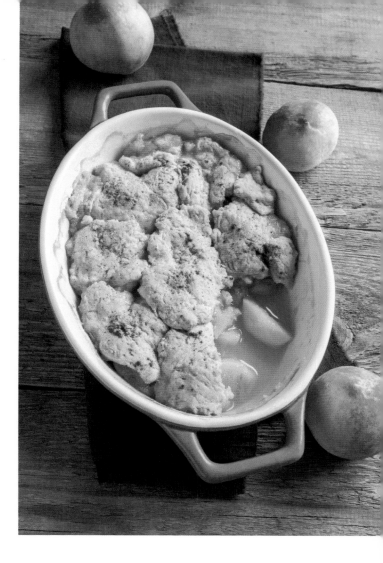

Filling
5 peaches, skinned / peeled,
pitted and sliced
3 Tbsp sugar
1 tsp tapioca flour (tapioca starch)
1/4 tsp cinnamon, ground
1/8 tsp nutmeg, ground
oil for the baking dish

Topping
120 ml almond flour
65g tapioca flour (tapioca starch)
1 1/2 tsp baking powder
60 ml almond milk, unsweetened
60 ml oil
1 tsp vanilla extract
1 Tbsp sugar

For Sprinkling (optional)
1 Tbsp sugar
1/2 tsp cinnamon, ground

Place sliced peaches, sugar, tapioca, cinnamon, and nutmeg in a bowl and mix well. Grease a baking dish with oil and spread the peach mixture in it.
Topping: combine almond flour, tapioca, baking powder, almond milk, oil, vanilla extract, and 1 tablespoon of sugar. Mix until smooth, then pour over the peaches.
If desired, mix 1 Tbsp of sugar with 1/2 tsp of cinnamon and sprinkle over the batter. Bake in a preheated oven at 190°C for 25 – 35 minutes. Do the toothpick test. Serve with vegan ice cream.

CHERRY PIE

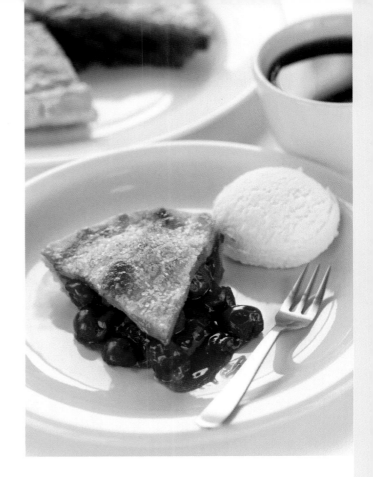

Crust
90g oat flour, gluten-free
160g rice flour
1 Tbsp tapioca flour (tapioca starch)
1/2 tsp salt
150g vegan margarine
2-3 Tbsp water

Filling
1 kg fresh cherries, stoned
1 Tbsp lemon juice
5 Tbsp maple syrup
3 Tbsp tapioca flour (tapioca starch)

Place washed and stoned cherries into a pot, add lemon juice, maple syrup, and tapioca and cook over medium heat for about 15 minutes until sauce has thickened. Let cool fully.

Put oat flour, rice flour, tapioca, and salt in a bowl and mix well. Add vegan margarine and work it evenly into the flour mixture. Add one Tbsp of water at a time and knead the dough well with your hands. Cut the dough in half, wrap both parts in cling film/plastic wrap and place in the fridge for 15 minutes.

Then place one half of the dough on baking paper and roll out to a circle, large enough to fill your pie dish. Lift and flip baking paper and dough into the dish. Remove the baking paper and align dough edges with the pie dish edges. Evenly pour the cooled cherries on the dough in the pie dish.

Place the other half of the dough on baking paper and roll out into a circle as well. Lift and flip the baking paper and dough on the cherry filling. Remove the baking paper and press down the edges of the dough using your fingers or a fork.

Bake in preheated oven at 190°C for 30-40 minutes and let cool completely before cutting. Sprinkle with coarse-grained sugar as desired and serve with a scoop of vanilla ice cream.

PUMPKIN PIE

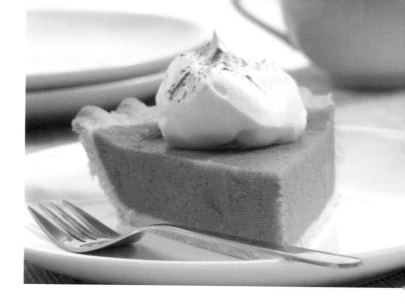

Crust
50g oat flour, gluten-free
75g rice flour
1/2 Tbsp tapioca flour/starch
1/4 tsp salt
75g vegan margarine
1-2 Tbsp water

Filling
450g pumpkin purée	salt	240 ml almond milk
150g sugar	30g tapioca flour/starch	1 tsp cinnamon, ground
1/2 tsp nutmeg, ground	pinch of cloves, ground	1/2 tsp ginger, ground

Wash and cut pumpkin in half. Remove the seeds with a spoon. Lightly salt the halves and place them, flesh facing down, on a baking tray covered with baking paper. Bake in a preheated oven at 200°C for 45 minutes. Then let the pumpkin cool down.

Put oat flour, rice flour, tapioca, and salt in a bowl and mix well. Add vegan margarine and work it evenly into the flour mixture. Add water one tablespoon at a time and knead the dough well with your hands. Wrap dough in cling film/plastic wrap and place in fridge for 15 minutes.

Place cooled dough on baking paper and roll out to a circle, large enough to fill your pie dish. Lift and flip baking paper and dough into the pie dish. Remove baking paper. Align edges of dough with the edges of the pie dish.

Spoon out 450g of baked pumpkin flesh, and place in a food processor. Add almond milk, sugar, tapioca, and spices and blend until smooth. Pour mixture evenly on dough in pie dish. Bake in preheated oven at 180°C for 45 minutes and let cool completely. Store pie in the refrigerator for several hours, preferably overnight. Serve with vegan whipped cream.

If pumpkin is left over, it can be frozen. If water forms after defrosting, drain the water.

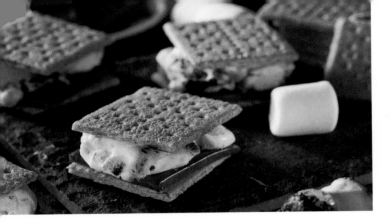

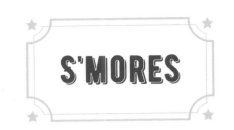

Graham Crackers

280g gluten-free flour
1/4 tsp salt
120g vegan margarine

1/2 tsp baking powder
1 tsp cinnamon, ground
3 Tbsp water

1/2 tsp baking soda
80g brown sugar
3 Tbsp maple syrup

vegan marshmallows

dark chocolate

Put gluten-free flour, baking powder, baking soda, salt, cinnamon, and sugar in bowl and mix well. Add vegan margarine and work it in nicely. Add water and maple syrup. Knead until you have a smooth dough. Wrap dough in cling film/plastic wrap and place in fridge for one hour.

On a floured work surface, divide dough into 4 parts and roll out each part separately with a rolling pin, roughly making squares about 5 mm thick. Make perfect squares by cutting the edges straight with a knife or pizza cutter. Finally, knead all leftover dough edges and roll them out into a square as well. Now use the knife or pizza cutter to divide all these perfect squares into smaller 5 cm squares. Prick the 5 cm squares several times with a fork. Place the squares on a baking tray covered with baking paper and bake in a preheated oven at 180°C for 5-10 minutes until the crackers turn light brown at the edges.

Skewer vegan marshmallows and roast them on a campfire or grill while turning them regularly (only suitable for large marshmallows). Alternatively, place the marshmallows in an aluminium tray and roast them on the grill rack, turning several times. Roasting without grill or campfire: Place marshmallows in an ovenproof dish and heat in the oven at 160°C for 8 minutes.

Assemble the S'mores: place one piece of dark chocolate on each graham cracker and one soft marshmallow on top. Top it off with another graham cracker, gently compress and enjoy.

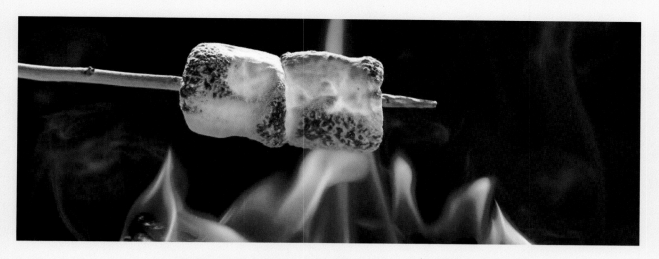

skewered marshmallows over a campfire

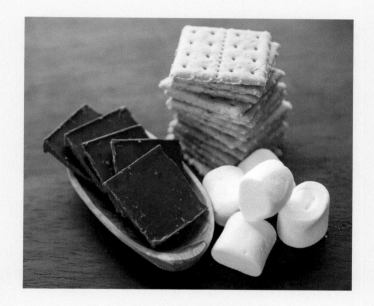

<u>s'mores ingredients</u>
graham crackers
marshmallows
dark chocolate

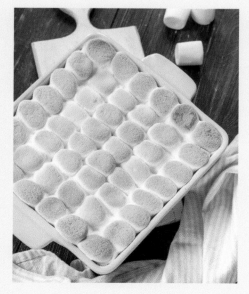

marshmallows from the oven

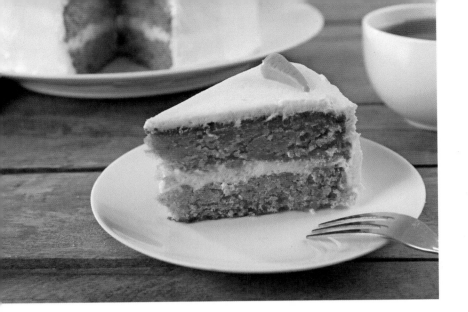

CARROT CAKE

150g sugar
180 ml oil
400g oat flour, gluten-free
1 tsp baking soda
1/2 tsp salt
1/2 tsp nutmeg, ground
120g walnuts, chopped

180 ml almond milk
1 Tbsp apple cider vinegar
1 tsp baking powder
1/2 tsp vanilla extract
2 tsp cinnamon, ground
6 carrots, medium-sized, finely grated
oil for the springform

Put sugar, almond milk, oil, and apple cider vinegar in a bowl and mix well. Add oat flour, baking powder, baking soda, vanilla extract, salt, cinnamon, and nutmeg and stir well until smooth. Then combine carrots and walnuts into the mixture.

Pour batter evenly into a pre-greased 26 cm springform pan lined with baking paper. Bake in a preheated oven at 180°C for about 50 minutes. Before ending the baking process, carry out a toothpick test and adjust baking time if needed. Once finished, remove from oven and allow to cool. When cool enough to touch, remove the ring from the cake and let it cool completely so that the frosting does not melt off.

In the meantime, prepare frosting (see frosting ingredients on page 53): Sieve icing sugar into a bowl, add all other frosting ingredients and beat with a hand mixer until mixture thickens into a frosting.

Cut the cooled cake into two equally thick layers by using a long knife and cutting horizontally down the middle. Remove the top layer. Frost the top of the bottom layer and replace the top layer. Now spread the frosting on the top and sides, coating the entire cake with frosting. Design the frosting and decorate as desired.

RED VELVET CAKE

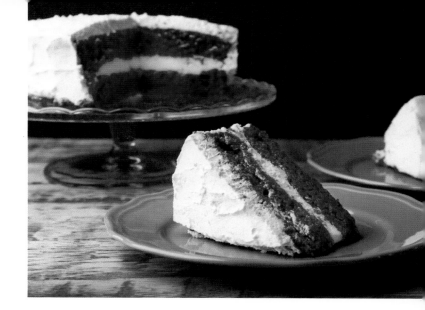

230 ml soy milk
1 Tbsp lemon juice
250g gluten-free flour
200g sugar
1 tsp baking soda
1/2 tsp salt
1 Tbsp unsweetened cocoa powder
1 tsp vanilla extract
80 ml oil
1 Tbsp apple cider vinegar
3 Tbsp vegan food colouring, red
oil for the springform

Frosting
400g icing sugar
55g vegan margarine, room temperature
3 Tbsp vegan cream cheese, room temperature
1 Tbsp lemon juice
1 tsp vanilla extract

Mix soy milk and lemon juice and let rest at room temperature for 5 minutes.
Sift flour into a bowl and mix with sugar, baking soda, salt, and cocoa powder. Add the soy milk and lemon juice mixture, vanilla extract, oil, apple cider vinegar, and red food colouring to the dry ingredients and whisk to a smooth batter.
Pour batter evenly into a pre-greased 26 cm springform pan lined with baking paper. Bake in a preheated oven at 180°C for 40 minutes. Before ending the baking process, carry out a toothpick test, adjust baking time if needed. Remove to cool once finished baking. When cool enough to touch, remove the ring from the cake and let it cool completely so that the frosting does not melt off.
In the meantime, prepare the frosting: Sieve icing sugar into a bowl, add all remaining frosting ingredients and beat with a hand mixer until the mixture thickens into a frosting.
Cut the cooled cake into two equally thick layers by using a long knife and cutting horizontally down the middle. Remove the top layer. Frost the top of the bottom layer and replace the top layer. Now spread the frosting on the top and sides, coating the entire cake with frosting. Design the frosting and decorate as desired.

Copyright © 2020 Annette Heringmann
ISBN Paperback: 978-1-7770099-5-3

SD International Inc. • Edmonton • Alberta • Canada
sd.international.inc@gmail.com

All rights reserved. No part of this publication may be reproduced, distributed, or transmitted in any form or by any means, including photocopying, recording, or other electronic or mechanical methods, without the prior written permission of the publisher, except in the case of brief quotations embodied in critical reviews and certain other non-commercial uses permitted by copyright law.

The author put forth her best effort to make this book a reality by bringing these recipes together. The information herein, i.e. the ingredients, suggestions, and directions are guidelines only. Different appliance brands, wattages, and temperatures will lead to slightly different outcomes. We recommend fully reading a recipe before starting it and to always use your best judgement. We disavow any and all responsibility for any and all adverse effects resulting from the use or misuse of the information provided in these recipes.

Neither the publisher nor the author is responsible for any adverse reaction to the ingredients contained in this book. Nor are they responsible for your specific health or allergy needs that may require medical supervision.

If you have any questions, comments, or just want to say hi, send an email to sd.international.inc@gmail.com.

Thank you

Printed in Germany
by Amazon Distribution
GmbH, Leipzig

18809855R00032